NAVIGATING WEIGHT LOSS

A Practical Guide to Weight Loss and Balanced Nutrition

Contents

1. INTRODUCTION TO WEIGHT LOSS AND NUTRITION

Losing weight is a goal that many individuals strive to achieve for various reasons, including improving overall health, enhancing self-confidence and increasing energy levels. One of the key pillars of achieving sustainable weight loss is understanding the intricate relationship between nutrition and the body's metabolic processes. Nutrition, as a crucial component, plays a fundamental role in not just shedding unwanted pounds but also in promoting overall well-being.

This introductory chapter aims to provide a comprehensive overview of the fundamental principles of weight loss and the significance of nutrition in this process. It will delve into the basics of how the body processes food, the role of calories and the impact of different nutrients on the body's composition and energy levels. By grasping these foundational concepts, individuals can make informed and effective choices regarding their dietary habits, leading to successful weight management and improved health outcomes.

Throughout this guide, we will explore evidence-based strategies for incorporating nutritious and balanced meal plans, the importance of mindful eating and how to develop sustainable lifestyle habits that support long-term weight management. Additionally, we will debunk common myths and misconceptions surrounding weight loss and nutrition, providing readers with accurate and practical information to facilitate their journey towards a healthier and more fulfilling lifestyle.

By delving into the principles of weight loss and nutrition, readers will gain valuable insights and tools to embark on a successful and sustainable weight loss journey that prioritizes both physical and mental well-being. With a focus on evidence-based practices and practical tips, this guide aims to empower individuals to make informed decisions and foster a positive relationship with food, leading to lasting transformations and improved overall quality of life.

a. Understanding the Basics of Weight Loss

Weight loss is the result of an imbalance between the number of calories consumed and the number of calories expended. This fundamental principle forms the basis of various weight loss strategies and programs. In essence, when the body expends more energy than it consumes, it taps into its stored energy reserves, leading to a reduction in body weight. However, achieving sustainable weight loss requires a comprehensive understanding of the factors that influence this intricate process.

This section will delve into the key components of weight loss, including the role of metabolism, the significance of calorie deficit and the impact of physical activity on overall energy expenditure. By comprehending these underlying mechanisms, individuals can make informed choices about their dietary habits and lifestyle modifications, facilitating a more effective and sustainable approach to weight management.

Furthermore, this section will highlight the importance of setting realistic and attainable weight loss goals, emphasizing the need for patience and perseverance throughout the journey. By establishing clear objectives and understanding the time and effort required to achieve them, individuals can cultivate a positive and resilient mindset, essential for long-term success in their weight loss endeavors.

By gaining a deeper understanding of the basics of weight loss, readers will be equipped with the knowledge and tools necessary to make informed decisions about their dietary and lifestyle choices. This knowledge will serve as a solid foundation for implementing effective strategies and sustainable practices that promote not only weight loss but also overall health and well-being.

b. Importance of Nutrition in Achieving Weight Loss Goals

Nutrition plays a pivotal role in the successful attainment of weight loss goals. While physical activity and exercise contribute to energy expenditure, the quality and composition of one's diet significantly impact the body's ability to shed excess weight and maintain a healthy balance. Understanding the importance of nutrition in this context is vital for designing an effective and sustainable weight loss plan.

This section will emphasize the role of nutrition in fueling the body with essential nutrients while simultaneously creating a calorie deficit necessary for weight loss. It will explore the significance of consuming whole, nutrient-dense foods that provide essential vitamins, minerals and antioxidants, fostering overall well-being and supporting the body's metabolic functions.

Moreover, the section will address the impact of macronutrients, such as carbohydrates, proteins and fats, on weight management, highlighting the importance of striking the right balance to support satiety, muscle retention and energy levels. It will also underscore the role of micronutrients in optimizing metabolic processes and promoting overall health, emphasizing the need for a diverse and well-rounded diet to ensure adequate nutrient intake.

Additionally, the section will delve into the concept of mindful eating, encouraging individuals to cultivate a conscious and intuitive approach to their dietary habits. By fostering a deeper understanding of hunger cues, portion control and food choices, individuals can develop a healthier relationship with food, thereby facilitating sustainable and long-term weight management.

By recognizing the critical role of nutrition in the context of weight loss, readers will be empowered to make informed and mindful choices about their dietary habits, ultimately fostering a healthier and more sustainable lifestyle. Through a comprehensive understanding of the impact of nutrition on overall well-being, individuals can establish a solid foundation for achieving and maintaining their weight loss goals, leading to improved physical health and enhanced quality of life.

2. ASSESSING YOUR CURRENT HEALTH AND GOALS

Before embarking on any weight loss journey, it is crucial to conduct a comprehensive assessment of your current health status and set realistic and achievable goals. This process serves as a critical foundation for developing a personalized and effective weight loss plan tailored to your individual needs and circumstances.

This section will guide you through the process of evaluating your current health, including assessing your body mass index (BMI), understanding your body composition and identifying any underlying health conditions that may impact your weight loss journey. By gaining a holistic understanding of your current health status, you can establish a clear starting point and identify any potential challenges or considerations that may need to be addressed.

Furthermore, this section will emphasize the importance of setting specific, measurable, achievable, relevant and time-bound (SMART) goals. It will provide practical guidance on how to set realistic and attainable weight loss targets that align with your personal preferences, lifestyle and overall health objectives. By establishing clear and meaningful goals, you can stay motivated and focused throughout your weight loss journey, increasing the likelihood of successful outcomes.

Moreover, the section will underscore the significance of seeking guidance from healthcare professionals, including physicians, nutritionists and fitness experts. By consulting with these professionals, you can gain valuable insights and recommendations tailored to your unique health profile, ensuring a safe and effective approach to your weight loss endeavors.

By conducting a comprehensive assessment of your current health status and setting clear and realistic goals, you will be better equipped to embark on a successful weight loss journey. This proactive approach will enable you to develop a customized and sustainable plan that addresses your specific needs and aspirations, leading to improved health outcomes and a positive transformation in your overall well-being.

a. Setting Realistic Weight Loss Goals

Body Mass Index (BMI) is a simple yet useful measure to assess whether an individual's weight is within a healthy range relative to their height. It serves as a starting point for understanding one's overall body composition and provides insight into potential health risks associated with weight.

To calculate your BMI, use the following formula:

BMI = (Weight in kilograms) / (Height in meters)^2

or

BMI = (Weight in pounds) / (Height in inches)^2 *703

Once you have calculated your BMI, you can interpret the results using the standard BMI categories:

- BMI below 18.5: Underweight

- BMI 18.5 to 24.9: Normal weight

- BMI 25.0 to 29.9: Overweight

- BMI 30.0 and above: Obesity

Understanding your BMI category can provide valuable insights into your weight status and potential health risks associated with being underweight, overweight, or obese. However, it's important to recognize that BMI is a general measurement and may not account for specific factors such as muscle mass or body composition. Therefore, it's advisable to consider other health indicators and consult with a healthcare professional for a comprehensive evaluation of your overall health status.

By determining your BMI, you can gain a preliminary understanding of your weight status and use this information as a basis for setting achievable weight management goals. Incorporating other health metrics alongside BMI can provide a more comprehensive view of your health and guide you in making informed decisions to achieve a healthier lifestyle.

b. Consulting with a Healthcare Professional

Setting realistic weight loss goals is crucial for maintaining motivation and ensuring long-term success on your weight loss journey. Unrealistic goals can lead to frustration and may even hamper your progress. Here are some key steps to setting achievable weight loss goals:

1. Consult a Healthcare Professional: Seek guidance from a healthcare provider or a registered dietitian to determine a healthy and realistic weight loss goal based on your BMI, health history and individual circumstances.

2. Be Specific and Measurable: Set clear and measurable goals, such as aiming to lose a specific number of pounds or inches over a designated period. Breaking down your overall goal into smaller, manageable targets can make it more achievable.

3. Consider a Realistic Timeframe: Establish a reasonable timeframe for achieving your weight loss goal. While it's natural to want rapid results, slow and steady weight loss is often more sustainable and healthier in the long run.

4. Focus on Health, Not Just Weight: Instead of solely focusing on the number on the scale, prioritize improving your overall health and well-being. Consider incorporating

goals related to increasing physical activity, improving dietary habits and enhancing overall fitness.

5. Set Behavioral Goals: Concentrate on developing healthy habits rather than solely focusing on outcomes. Examples include committing to a regular exercise routine, increasing vegetable intake, or reducing portion sizes.

6. Track Your Progress: Keep a record of your progress, including weight measurements, dietary changes and exercise routines. Regularly monitoring your progress can help you stay motivated and adjust your goals accordingly.

7. Stay Realistic and Flexible: Recognize that weight loss progress may fluctuate and plateaus are common. Be prepared to adjust your goals if necessary and stay committed to long-term lifestyle changes rather than short-term fixes.

8. Celebrate Milestones: Acknowledge and celebrate your achievements along the way, whether it's reaching a certain weight milestone or successfully sticking to your exercise routine. Celebrating your progress can help maintain motivation and keep you on track toward your ultimate weight loss goal.

By setting realistic and achievable weight loss goals, you can create a sustainable plan that promotes a healthier lifestyle and improves your overall well-being. It's important to approach weight loss as a gradual and holistic process, incorporating healthy habits that can be maintained in the long term for lasting results.

3. FUNDAMENTALS OF CALORIES AND ENERGY BALANCE

Understanding the fundamentals of calories and energy balance is essential for effective weight management. The concept of energy balance revolves around the principle that the energy consumed through food and beverages should be balanced with the energy expended through physical activity and bodily functions. Here's a breakdown of the key components:

1. Caloric Intake: This refers to the number of calories consumed through food and beverages. Different foods contain varying amounts of calories and it's important to be mindful of portion sizes and the overall quality of your diet.

2. Caloric Expenditure: This encompasses the energy your body uses for basic physiological functions (basal metabolic rate), physical activity and the energy required for the digestion and absorption of food (thermic effect of food).

3. Energy Balance Equation: This equation represents the balance between caloric intake and caloric expenditure. A positive energy balance occurs when you consume more calories than you burn, leading to weight gain. Conversely, a negative energy balance results in weight loss as the body taps into stored energy reserves to make up for the deficit.

4. Metabolic Rate: Basal metabolic rate (BMR) is the number of calories your body needs to maintain basic physiological functions at rest, such as breathing, circulation and cell production. Understanding your BMR can help you determine an appropriate calorie intake for weight loss or maintenance.

5. Factors Affecting Energy Balance: Various factors can influence energy balance, including genetics, age, gender, body composition, hormone levels and physical activity levels. It's important to consider these factors when designing a personalized weight management plan.

By comprehending the fundamentals of calories and energy balance, you can make informed decisions about your dietary choices and physical activity levels to achieve and maintain a healthy weight. Balancing caloric intake with caloric expenditure is key to successful weight management and overall well-being. It's essential to focus on creating a sustainable lifestyle that promotes a healthy energy balance and supports long-term health goals.

a. Understanding Caloric Intake and Expenditure

Understanding caloric intake and expenditure is crucial for effective weight management and maintaining overall health. Here's a breakdown of each component:

1. Caloric Intake:

- Food Composition: Different foods contain varying amounts of calories. It's essential to focus on a balanced diet that includes nutrient-dense whole foods, such as fruits, vegetables, whole grains, lean proteins and healthy fats.

- Portion Control: Pay attention to portion sizes to ensure that you're not consuming more calories than your body needs. Mindful eating practices can help you develop a healthy relationship with food and promote better portion control.

- Nutritional Labels: Read nutritional labels to understand the caloric content and serving sizes of packaged foods. This can help you make informed decisions about your food choices.

2. Caloric Expenditure:

- Basal Metabolic Rate (BMR): BMR represents the number of calories your body needs to maintain basic physiological functions at rest. Factors such as age, weight, height and gender influence your BMR. Calculating your

BMR can provide insights into the minimum number of calories your body requires daily.

- Physical Activity: Regular exercise and physical activity contribute to additional caloric expenditure. Engaging in both cardiovascular activities and strength training can help boost your overall energy expenditure and support weight loss or maintenance.

- Non-Exercise Activity Thermogenesis (NEAT): NEAT encompasses the energy expended during non-exercise activities, such as walking, fidgeting and daily chores. Increasing NEAT can contribute to overall caloric expenditure.

Understanding the balance between caloric intake and expenditure is crucial for achieving and maintaining a healthy weight. By focusing on a balanced diet, practicing portion control and incorporating regular physical activity into your routine, you can create a sustainable lifestyle that supports your overall health and well-being. It's important to find a personalized approach that works best for you and promotes a healthy energy balance.

b. Calculating Basal Metabolic Rate (BMR) and Total Daily Energy Expenditure (TDEE)

Calculating your Basal Metabolic Rate (BMR) and Total Daily Energy Expenditure (TDEE) can provide valuable insights into the number of calories your body needs to maintain its current weight and the number of calories required to support your daily activity level. Here's how you can estimate both:

1. Basal Metabolic Rate (BMR):

   - For men: BMR = 88.362 + (13.397 x weight in kg) + (4.799 x height in cm) - (5.677 x age in years)

   - For women: BMR = 447.593 + (9.247 x weight in kg) + (3.098 x height in cm) - (4.330 x age in years)

2. Total Daily Energy Expenditure (TDEE):

   - Sedentary (little or no exercise): BMR x 1.2

   - Lightly active (light exercise/sports 1-3 days a week): BMR x 1.375

   - Moderately active (moderate exercise/sports 3-5 days a week): BMR x 1.55

   - Very active (hard exercise/sports 6-7 days a week): BMR x 1.725

- Super active (very hard exercise and a physical job): BMR x 1.9

Using these formulas, you can estimate your BMR and TDEE, which can serve as a starting point for understanding your daily caloric needs. It's important to note that these calculations provide rough estimates and individual variations exist based on factors such as body composition, genetics and hormone levels. Adjustments may be necessary based on your personal experience and progress.

Understanding your BMR and TDEE can help you make informed decisions about calorie intake and expenditure, enabling you to create a personalized nutrition and exercise plan that supports your health and fitness goals. Keep in mind that these calculations serve as guidelines and consulting with a healthcare professional or registered dietitian can provide further insights and guidance tailored to your specific needs and objectives.

4. ESSENTIAL NUTRIENTS FOR WEIGHT LOSS

Essential nutrients play a vital role in supporting weight loss efforts while ensuring optimal health and well-being. When focusing on weight loss, it's crucial to prioritize nutrient-dense foods that provide essential vitamins, minerals and other key nutrients. Here are some essential nutrients that can aid in weight loss:

1. Protein: Incorporating adequate protein into your diet can promote satiety, help preserve lean muscle mass and support metabolism. Good sources of protein include lean meats, poultry, fish, legumes, tofu and dairy products.

2. Fiber: High-fiber foods can help control hunger and promote feelings of fullness, leading to reduced calorie intake. Additionally, fiber supports digestive health and can aid in regulating blood sugar levels. Include whole grains, fruits, vegetables, nuts and seeds in your diet to increase your fiber intake.

3. Healthy Fats: Consuming healthy fats in moderation can contribute to satiety and help you feel satisfied after meals. Sources of healthy fats include avocados, nuts, seeds and olive oil. These fats also play a role in supporting various bodily functions and promoting overall health.

4. Complex Carbohydrates: Opt for complex carbohydrates, such as whole grains, fruits and vegetables, which provide sustained energy and help stabilize blood sugar levels. These foods can keep you feeling full for longer periods, reducing the likelihood of overeating or snacking on unhealthy options.

5. Vitamins and Minerals: Essential vitamins and minerals, such as vitamin D, calcium, iron and magnesium, are crucial for overall health and can support various metabolic processes in the body. Consuming a diverse range of fruits, vegetables and whole foods can help ensure you meet your daily requirements for these nutrients.

6. Hydration: While not a traditional nutrient, staying adequately hydrated is crucial for supporting weight loss. Drinking plenty of water can help control appetite, boost metabolism and improve overall energy levels. Aim to consume water throughout the day and limit sugary beverages and excessive caffeine intake.

Incorporating these essential nutrients into your diet can support your weight loss goals while providing your body with the necessary elements for optimal functioning and overall health. Strive for a balanced and varied diet that includes a wide range of nutrient-dense foods to promote sustainable weight loss and long-term well-being. Additionally, consult with a healthcare professional or registered dietitian to develop a personalized nutrition plan that meets your specific dietary needs and weight loss objectives.

a. Macronutrients: Carbohydrates, Proteins and Fats

Macronutrients, including carbohydrates, proteins and fats, are essential components of a balanced diet that play a critical role in supporting various bodily functions and promoting overall health. Understanding the role of each macronutrient can help you make informed dietary choices to support your weight loss goals. Here's an overview of each macronutrient:

1. Carbohydrates:

- Carbohydrates are the primary source of energy for the body. They are classified into two main types: complex carbohydrates (found in whole grains, vegetables and legumes) and simple carbohydrates (found in fruits and refined sugars).

- Focus on consuming complex carbohydrates, which provide sustained energy, fiber, vitamins and minerals. These can help you feel fuller for longer periods, reducing the likelihood of overeating and promoting stable blood sugar levels.

2. Proteins:

- Proteins are essential for building and repairing tissues, supporting muscle growth and regulating various metabolic processes. Good sources of protein include lean meats, poultry, fish, eggs, dairy products, legumes and plant-based protein sources like tofu and tempeh.

- Including adequate protein in your diet can promote satiety, reduce cravings and help preserve lean muscle mass, which is essential for supporting overall metabolic health during weight loss.

3. Fats:

- Dietary fats play a crucial role in providing energy, supporting cell growth, protecting organs and helping the body absorb fat-soluble vitamins. Healthy fat sources include avocados, nuts, seeds, olive oil, fatty fish and plant-based oils.

- Incorporate unsaturated fats, such as monounsaturated and polyunsaturated fats, while limiting the intake of saturated and Tran's fats. Prioritizing healthy fats can help you feel satisfied after meals and support various bodily functions without promoting weight gain.

Balancing your intake of carbohydrates, proteins and fats is key to maintaining a well-rounded and nutritious diet. Opt for whole, unprocessed foods and be mindful of portion sizes to ensure that you're meeting your nutritional needs while effectively managing your caloric intake. Consulting with a registered dietitian can provide personalized guidance on how to incorporate the right balance of macronutrients into your diet to support your weight loss goals and overall health.

b. Micronutrients: Vitamins and Minerals

Micronutrients, including vitamins and minerals, are essential for supporting various physiological functions, promoting overall health and aiding in the process of weight loss. These vital nutrients play key roles in metabolism, immune function, energy production and the maintenance of bone and tissue health. Here's an overview of some important vitamins and minerals:

1. Vitamins:

- Vitamin A: Supports vision, immune function and skin health. Good sources include carrots, sweet potatoes, spinach and dairy products.

- Vitamin C: Supports immune function, wound healing and the absorption of iron. Found in citrus fruits, bell peppers, strawberries and leafy greens.

- Vitamin D: Essential for bone health, immune function and the regulation of calcium levels. Sunlight exposure, fatty fish and fortified dairy products are good sources.

- Vitamin E: Acts as an antioxidant and supports skin health and immune function. Nuts, seeds and vegetable oils are good sources of vitamin E.

2. Minerals:

- Calcium: Essential for bone health, muscle function and nerve transmission. Dairy products, leafy greens and fortified foods are good sources.

- Iron: Necessary for oxygen transport, energy production and immune function. Found in red meat, poultry, beans and fortified grains.

- Magnesium: Supports muscle and nerve function, blood sugar regulation and bone health. Nuts, seeds, whole grains and leafy greens are good sources.

- Potassium: Aids in maintaining healthy blood pressure, nerve function and muscle contractions. Bananas, potatoes and leafy greens are good sources of potassium.

Incorporating a variety of fruits, vegetables, whole grains, lean proteins and dairy products into your diet can help ensure that you're obtaining an adequate intake of essential vitamins and minerals. A balanced and diverse diet that includes a wide range of nutrient-dense foods can help support your weight loss efforts while promoting overall health and well-being. If you have specific dietary concerns or restrictions, consult with a healthcare professional or registered dietitian to develop a personalized nutrition plan that meets your individual needs and goals.

c. Importance of Fiber in Weight Management

Fiber plays a crucial role in weight management and overall well-being. It is a type of carbohydrate that the body cannot digest and it comes in two forms: soluble and insoluble. Both forms offer various health benefits, particularly when it comes to weight management. Here are some reasons why fiber is essential for supporting weight loss:

1. Promotes Satiety: Fiber-rich foods help you feel full and satisfied for longer periods, reducing overall food intake and preventing overeating. This can be especially beneficial in controlling cravings and managing portion sizes, ultimately supporting weight loss efforts.

2. Regulates Digestion: Fiber aids in regulating bowel movements and promoting healthy digestion. By preventing constipation and promoting regularity, fiber supports a healthy gut microbiome, which is linked to improved metabolic health and weight management.

3. Stabilizes Blood Sugar Levels: Soluble fiber can slow down the absorption of sugar, helping to stabilize blood sugar levels. This can prevent rapid spikes and crashes in blood sugar, which can lead to cravings and overeating, particularly of sugary and high-calorie foods.

4. Lowers Cholesterol Levels: Certain types of soluble fiber can help reduce levels of LDL (bad) cholesterol, which is linked to an increased risk of heart disease. By incorporating fiber-rich foods into your diet, you can support heart health while working towards your weight loss goals.

5. Supports Gut Health: Fiber serves as a prebiotic, promoting the growth of beneficial bacteria in the gut. A healthy gut microbiome is associated with improved digestion, metabolism and overall immune function, all of which contribute to better weight management and overall health.

To increase your fiber intake, incorporate a variety of whole grains, fruits, vegetables, legumes, nuts and seeds into your daily diet. Gradually increasing your fiber intake and staying adequately hydrated can help prevent any potential digestive discomfort. As part of a balanced diet and healthy lifestyle, fiber can be a valuable asset in your weight management journey, promoting overall health and well-being.

5. DESIGNING A BALANCED AND SUSTAINABLE MEAL PLAN

Designing a balanced and sustainable meal plan is crucial for achieving and maintaining a healthy weight while ensuring that your body receives the necessary nutrients for optimal functioning. Here are some key considerations to keep in mind when creating your meal plan:

1. Incorporate a Variety of Nutrient-Dense Foods: Include a diverse range of fruits, vegetables, whole grains, lean proteins and healthy fats to ensure that you're receiving a wide spectrum of essential vitamins, minerals and antioxidants.

2. Prioritize Portion Control: Be mindful of portion sizes to avoid overeating and unnecessary calorie consumption. Using smaller plates, bowls and containers can help manage portion sizes and prevent overindulgence.

3. Emphasize Whole Foods: Choose whole, unprocessed foods over refined and processed options. Whole foods contain higher amounts of nutrients, fiber and beneficial compounds, supporting overall health and satiety.

4. Plan Meals around Protein and Fiber: Center your meals around lean protein sources and high-fiber foods to promote satiety, stabilize blood sugar levels and support

muscle maintenance. Incorporate a variety of plant-based and animal-based protein options into your meal plan.

5. Include Healthy Fats: Incorporate sources of healthy fats, such as avocados, nuts, seeds and olive oil, to promote satiety and support various bodily functions. Healthy fats can help you feel satisfied after meals and reduce the likelihood of unhealthy snacking.

6. Stay Hydrated: Include plenty of water throughout the day and limit the consumption of sugary beverages. Staying adequately hydrated can support digestion, promote satiety and help prevent unnecessary calorie intake.

7. Plan Ahead and Prep Meals: Plan your meals in advance and consider meal prepping to ensure that you have healthy options readily available. This can help you avoid the temptation of unhealthy convenience foods and make it easier to stick to your meal plan.

8. Practice Mindful Eating: Pay attention to hunger and fullness cues and eat slowly to fully enjoy and savor your meals. Mindful eating can help prevent overeating and promote a healthier relationship with food.

By designing a balanced and sustainable meal plan that incorporates these principles, you can support your weight management goals while promoting overall health and well-being. Consult with a registered dietitian or nutritionist to create a personalized meal plan that aligns with your dietary preferences, lifestyle and specific health needs.

a. Portion Control and Meal Timing

Portion control and meal timing are crucial aspects of a balanced and effective weight management plan. By paying attention to the size of your portions and the timing of your meals, you can better regulate your caloric intake, support healthy digestion and manage your hunger levels. Here are some tips for incorporating portion control and meal timing into your daily routine:

1. Understand Serving Sizes: Familiarize yourself with standard serving sizes for different food groups. Use measuring tools, such as cups, spoons and food scales, to accurately portion your meals and snacks.

2. Use Smaller Plates and Bowls: Opt for smaller dishware to create the illusion of larger portions while controlling the actual amount of food you consume. This can help prevent overeating and promote better portion control.

3. Fill Half Your Plate with Vegetables: Make vegetables the focal point of your meals by filling at least half of your plate with a colorful variety of nutrient-dense vegetables. This can help you feel full while ensuring you receive essential vitamins, minerals and fiber.

4. Practice the Plate Method: Divide your plate into sections, allocating appropriate portions for protein, whole

grains and vegetables. This method can guide you in creating well-balanced meals that support portion control and overall nutrition.

5. Eat Mindfully: Pay attention to hunger and fullness cues while eating. Eat slowly, savor your food and avoid distractions, such as screens or multitasking, to fully engage with the eating experience and prevent overeating.

6. Establish Regular Meal Times: Aim to establish regular meal times and stick to a consistent eating schedule. This can help regulate your metabolism and prevent excessive snacking or overindulgence during irregular eating patterns.

7. Include Healthy Snacks: Plan nutritious snacks between meals to prevent extreme hunger and overeating during main meals. Opt for snacks that combine protein, healthy fats and fiber to help keep you satisfied and energized throughout the day.

8. Avoid Late-Night Eating: Limit your food intake in the evening and avoid heavy meals before bedtime. Allow sufficient time between your last meal and bedtime to support proper digestion and promote better sleep quality.

By incorporating portion control and mindful meal timing into your daily routine, you can develop healthier eating habits that support your weight management goals and promote overall well-being. Remember that balance and moderation are key and consulting with a registered dietitian can provide personalized guidance on portion control strategies and meal timing that align with your specific dietary needs and lifestyle.

b. Incorporating Whole Foods and Healthy Fats

Incorporating whole foods and healthy fats into your diet is essential for supporting weight management, promoting overall health and ensuring you receive a well-rounded and nutritious diet. Whole foods are rich in essential nutrients, including vitamins, minerals and antioxidants, while healthy fats provide energy and support various bodily functions. Here are some tips for incorporating whole foods and healthy fats into your daily meals:

1. Choose Whole Grains: Opt for whole grains such as quinoa, brown rice, barley and oats, which are rich in fiber and essential nutrients. Whole grains can help you feel full and satisfied, supporting healthy digestion and promoting stable energy levels.

2. Load Up on Vegetables and Fruits: Include a colorful variety of vegetables and fruits in your meals and snacks. These nutrient-dense foods provide essential vitamins, minerals and antioxidants, while also adding flavor and texture to your diet.

3. Incorporate Lean Protein Sources: Choose lean protein sources such as poultry, fish, legumes and tofu to support muscle maintenance and promote satiety. These protein-rich foods can help you feel full for longer periods and prevent excessive snacking.

4. Include Healthy Fats: Incorporate sources of healthy fats, including avocados, nuts, seeds and olive oil, in your diet. Healthy fats can help you feel satisfied after meals, support brain health and promote the absorption of fat-soluble vitamins.

5. Add Fatty Fish to Your Diet: Include fatty fish such as salmon, mackerel and trout, which are rich in omega-3 fatty acids. These essential fats are beneficial for heart health, cognitive function and overall well-being.

6. Use Natural Sweeteners: Opt for natural sweeteners like honey, maple syrup and dates, which provide a touch of sweetness while also offering some beneficial nutrients. Limit the use of refined sugars and processed sweeteners in your diet.

7. Snack on Nuts and Seeds: Incorporate a variety of nuts and seeds, such as almonds, walnuts, chia seeds and flaxseeds, into your snacks and meals. These nutrient-dense foods can provide a satisfying crunch while offering essential nutrients and healthy fats.

8. Cook with Healthy Oils: Use healthy oils such as olive oil, avocado oil and coconut oil for cooking and dressing your meals. These oils can add flavor to your dishes while

providing essential fatty acids and supporting overall health.

By incorporating whole foods and healthy fats into your daily diet, you can create a well-rounded and nutritious meal plan that supports your weight management goals and promotes overall well-being. Be mindful of portion sizes and balance your macronutrient intake to ensure that you're meeting your nutritional needs while effectively managing your caloric intake. Additionally, consulting with a registered dietitian can provide personalized guidance on how to incorporate whole foods and healthy fats into your diet to support your specific dietary preferences and health objectives.

c. Meal Prepping and Planning for Success

Meal prepping and planning are valuable strategies for achieving success in your weight management journey. By preparing and organizing your meals in advance, you can make healthier food choices, save time and avoid the temptation of unhealthy options. Here are some tips for effective meal prepping and planning:

1. Set Aside Time for Planning: Dedicate a specific time each week to plan your meals and create a detailed grocery list based on your meal plan. This can help you stay organized and ensure that you have all the necessary ingredients on hand.

2. Choose Balanced Recipes: Look for recipes that incorporate a balance of macronutrients and include a variety of whole foods, lean proteins and colorful vegetables. Select recipes that are easy to prepare and can be stored and reheated easily.

3. Prepare Meals in Bulk: Cook large batches of meals, such as soups, stews and grains that can be portioned and stored for future use. Divide the meals into individual containers to grab and go throughout the week.

4. Utilize Proper Storage Containers: Invest in high-quality, airtight containers that are suitable for storing different

types of food. Opt for containers that are microwave and freezer-safe to make reheating and preserving meals more convenient.

5. Include Snacks and Healthy Options: Prepare healthy snacks, such as cut fruits, vegetables and nuts, to have readily available when hunger strikes. Having nutritious options readily accessible can prevent you from reaching for processed or high-calorie snacks.

6. Label and Date Your Meals: Label each container with the name of the meal and the date it was prepared to ensure that you consume the meals within a safe timeframe. This can help you keep track of the freshness of your prepared meals.

7. Stay Flexible and Experiment: Be open to trying new recipes and ingredients to keep your meals exciting and flavorful. Rotate your meal options regularly to prevent boredom and maintain motivation to stick to your meal plan.

8. Create a Realistic Schedule: Plan your meals based on your weekly schedule and lifestyle. Consider your busiest days and prepare simpler meals or plan for leftovers on those days to avoid the need for last-minute unhealthy food choices.

By implementing effective meal prepping and planning strategies, you can set yourself up for success in achieving your weight management goals. Consistency and organization are key and with practice, meal prepping can become a sustainable and time-saving habit that supports your overall health and well-being. If you need further guidance or personalized meal planning advice, consult with a registered dietitian or nutritionist to develop a meal plan that aligns with your specific dietary needs and weight management objectives.

6. STRATEGIES FOR SUCCESSFUL WEIGHT LOSS

Achieving successful weight loss involves a combination of healthy lifestyle practices, mindful eating habits and regular physical activity. Here are some effective strategies to help you reach your weight loss goals:

1. Set Realistic Goals: Establish achievable and measurable weight loss goals that are realistic and sustainable over the long term. Break down your goals into smaller milestones to track your progress and stay motivated.

2. Create a Balanced Meal Plan: Develop a well-balanced meal plan that includes a variety of nutrient-dense foods, such as fruits, vegetables, lean proteins, whole grains and healthy fats. Focus on portion control and mindful eating to manage your caloric intake.

3. Practice Portion Control: Be mindful of portion sizes and use smaller plates and bowls to control your food portions. Pay attention to hunger and fullness cues to prevent overeating and unnecessary calorie consumption.

4. Incorporate Regular Exercise: Engage in regular physical activity, including cardiovascular exercises, strength training and flexibility exercises, to support your weight loss

journey. Find activities you enjoy to make exercise a sustainable part of your routine.

5. Stay Hydrated: Drink an adequate amount of water throughout the day to stay hydrated and support overall bodily functions. Sometimes, thirst can be mistaken for hunger, so staying hydrated can help prevent unnecessary snacking.

6. Get Sufficient Sleep: Aim for at least 7-9 hours of quality sleep each night to support your metabolism, energy levels and overall well-being. Prioritize a consistent sleep schedule and create a relaxing bedtime routine to promote better sleep quality.

7. Practice Mindful Eating: Pay attention to your eating habits and practice mindful eating by savoring each bite, chewing slowly and avoiding distractions during meals. This can help you appreciate food more and prevent overeating.

8. Manage Stress Levels: Find healthy ways to manage stress, such as meditation, yoga, deep breathing exercises, or engaging in hobbies you enjoy. High stress levels can contribute to emotional eating and hinder your weight loss efforts.

9. Seek Social Support: Surround yourself with a supportive network of friends, family, or a community group that shares your health and wellness goals. Sharing your journey with others can provide motivation, accountability and encouragement.

10. Monitor Your Progress: Keep track of your food intake, exercise routine and weight loss progress to assess your results and make necessary adjustments to your plan. Celebrate your achievements along the way, no matter how small.

By implementing these strategies and making healthy lifestyle choices, you can create a sustainable approach to weight loss that supports your overall health and well-being. Remember that every individual's journey is unique, so find the strategies that work best for you and consult with a healthcare professional or a registered dietitian for personalized guidance and support along the way.

a. The Role of Physical Activity in Weight Management

Physical activity plays a crucial role in weight management by helping to create a calorie deficit, promoting fat loss and improving overall health and well-being. Incorporating regular exercise into your routine can have a significant impact on your weight loss journey. Here's how physical activity contributes to effective weight management:

1. Calorie Expenditure: Engaging in physical activity helps you burn calories, which is essential for creating a calorie deficit and promoting weight loss. Combining regular exercise with a healthy diet can help you achieve a sustainable and healthy rate of weight loss.

2. Increased Metabolic Rate: Regular physical activity can help boost your metabolic rate, allowing your body to burn more calories throughout the day. This can be especially beneficial for weight maintenance and preventing weight regain after losing weight.

3. Preservation of Lean Muscle Mass: Incorporating resistance training and strength exercises into your routine can help preserve and build lean muscle mass. This is important for maintaining a higher metabolic rate, as muscle tissue burns more calories at rest than fat tissue.

4. Improved Cardiovascular Health: Physical activity supports cardiovascular health by strengthening the heart muscle, improving circulation and reducing the risk of cardiovascular diseases. A healthy cardiovascular system can enhance your ability to engage in more intense physical activities, further supporting your weight management efforts.

5. Enhanced Mood and Mental Well-Being: Exercise has been shown to improve mood, reduce stress and alleviate symptoms of anxiety and depression. By promoting overall mental well-being, regular physical activity can help reduce emotional eating and improve adherence to healthy lifestyle habits.

6. Regulation of Appetite and Hormones: Physical activity can help regulate appetite hormones, such as ghrelin and leptin, which play a role in hunger and satiety. Regular exercise can help control cravings and prevent overeating, contributing to better weight management.

7. Bone Health and Strength: Weight-bearing exercises, such as walking, running and resistance training, can help improve bone density and reduce the risk of osteoporosis. This is particularly important for overall health and mobility, especially as you age.

To maximize the benefits of physical activity for weight management, aim for a combination of cardiovascular exercises, strength training and flexibility exercises. Find activities you enjoy and can maintain in the long term to create a sustainable exercise routine that supports your weight loss goals and overall well-being. If you have any health concerns or specific fitness goals, consult with a healthcare professional or a certified fitness trainer to develop a safe and effective exercise plan tailored to your individual needs.

b. Mindful Eating and Behavior Modification Techniques

Mindful eating and behavior modification techniques are valuable strategies for promoting healthy eating habits, preventing overeating and supporting long-term weight management. By incorporating these techniques into your daily routine, you can develop a healthier relationship with food and make more conscious dietary choices. Here's how to integrate mindful eating and behavior modification techniques into your lifestyle:

1. Practice Mindful Eating:

  - Eat slowly and savor each bite to fully appreciate the flavors and textures of your food.

  - Pay attention to hunger and fullness cues to avoid overeating and promote better portion control.

  - Minimize distractions during meals, such as television or electronic devices, to focus on the sensory experience of eating.

  - Listen to your body's signals and stop eating when you feel comfortably full.

2. Keep a Food Journal:

  - Track your daily food intake, including portion sizes and meal times, to increase awareness of your eating habits and patterns.

- Note any emotional triggers or environmental cues that may lead to unhealthy eating behaviors.

- Review your food journal regularly to identify areas for improvement and celebrate your progress.

3. Identify Emotional Triggers:

- Recognize emotional triggers that may lead to stress eating or unhealthy food choices.

- Find alternative coping mechanisms, such as engaging in physical activity, practicing relaxation techniques, or seeking social support, to manage emotional distress without turning to food.

4. Create a Supportive Environment:

- Surround yourself with a supportive network of friends and family who encourage healthy eating habits and a positive body image.

- Limit the presence of unhealthy foods in your home and workplace to reduce temptation and promote healthier food choices.

5. Set Realistic Goals and Rewards:

- Establish achievable and measurable goals for your weight management journey.

- Reward yourself for reaching milestones with non-food-related incentives, such as a relaxing day at the spa, a new book, or a fun activity you enjoy.

6. Practice Stress Management:

- Incorporate stress management techniques, such as meditation, deep breathing exercises, or yoga, into your daily routine to reduce stress levels and prevent stress-related eating.

By integrating mindful eating practices and behavior modification techniques into your lifestyle, you can develop a healthier relationship with food, improve your eating behaviors and support sustainable weight management. These strategies can help you become more attuned to your body's needs and make conscious choices that align with your overall health and wellness goals. If you need additional guidance or support, consider consulting with a registered dietitian, therapist, or healthcare professional to develop a personalized plan that addresses your specific needs and challenges.

c. Coping with Cravings and Emotional Eating

Coping with cravings and emotional eating is essential for maintaining a healthy relationship with food and supporting successful weight management. By implementing effective strategies to manage cravings and address emotional triggers, you can develop healthier eating habits and make mindful dietary choices. Here are some techniques to help you cope with cravings and emotional eating:

1. Identify Triggers and Patterns:

   - Recognize the situations, emotions, or environments that trigger cravings or emotional eating episodes.

   - Keep a journal to track your cravings and note any emotional or situational patterns that may contribute to overeating.

2. Practice Mindfulness and Awareness:

   - Engage in mindful eating practices to become more conscious of your food choices and eating behaviors.

   - Pause and assess your hunger levels before reaching for food and consider whether you are eating out of hunger or in response to an emotional trigger.

3. Find Healthy Alternatives:

- Substitute unhealthy snacks with nutritious alternatives, such as fruits, vegetables, or nuts, to satisfy cravings without consuming excessive calories or processed foods.

- Opt for foods that are high in fiber and protein to promote satiety and prevent overeating.

4. Develop Healthy Coping Mechanisms:

- Find alternative ways to manage stress and emotions, such as engaging in physical activity, practicing relaxation techniques, or pursuing hobbies that bring you joy and fulfillment.

- Seek support from friends, family, or a therapist to address underlying emotional issues and develop effective coping strategies.

5. Create a Supportive Environment:

- Surround yourself with a supportive network of individuals who encourage healthy behaviors and provide positive reinforcement for your efforts to manage cravings and emotional eating.

- Communicate your needs and challenges to loved ones and seek their understanding and support in your journey toward healthier eating habits.

6. Plan Balanced Meals and Snacks:

- Incorporate balanced meals and snacks into your daily routine to prevent extreme hunger and reduce the likelihood of impulsive and unhealthy food choices.

- Include a variety of nutrient-dense foods, such as fruits, vegetables, lean proteins and healthy fats, to support overall health and well-being.

By implementing these coping strategies, you can develop healthier ways to manage cravings and emotional eating, fostering a more balanced and mindful approach to food and nutrition. If you find it challenging to overcome these behaviors on your own, consider seeking guidance from a registered dietitian, therapist, or healthcare professional, who can provide personalized support and guidance tailored to your specific needs and goals.

7. COMMON DIET PLANS AND THEIR EFFICACY

Various diet plans have gained popularity over the years, each with its unique approach to weight loss and overall health. While the efficacy of these diets can vary based on individual needs and preferences, here are some common diet plans and a brief overview of their general principles and potential efficacy:

1. Mediterranean Diet:

- Emphasizes the consumption of fruits, vegetables, whole grains, legumes, nuts and olive oil while limiting red meat and processed foods.

- Research suggests that the Mediterranean diet may promote heart health, weight management and overall well-being due to its focus on nutrient-dense foods and healthy fats.

2. Ketogenic Diet:

- Involves a high-fat, low-carbohydrate eating plan that aims to shift the body into a state of ketosis, where it burns fat for energy.

- While the ketogenic diet may lead to rapid weight loss, its long-term sustainability and potential health risks have raised concerns among some health professionals.

3. Paleo Diet:

- Advocates the consumption of foods believed to have been available to humans during the Paleolithic era, such as lean meats, fish, fruits, vegetables, nuts and seeds, while excluding grains, dairy and processed foods.

- While some people report weight loss and improved overall health on the Paleo diet, critics highlight potential nutritional deficiencies and the restrictive nature of the diet.

4. Vegetarian and Vegan Diets:

- Eliminate or limit the consumption of animal products, with vegetarian diets allowing for some animal-derived foods like dairy and eggs, while vegan diets exclude all animal products.

- Vegetarian and vegan diets can be effective for weight management and may offer various health benefits when properly planned to ensure adequate intake of essential nutrients like protein, iron and B vitamins.

5. DASH Diet:

- Focuses on consuming fruits, vegetables, whole grains, lean proteins and low-fat dairy while limiting foods high in saturated fats, sugar and sodium.

- The DASH diet is known for its effectiveness in lowering blood pressure and promoting heart health, making it a beneficial option for individuals looking to improve their overall cardiovascular well-being.

6. Intermittent Fasting:

- Involves alternating periods of fasting and eating, with various intermittent fasting methods, such as the 16/8 method or the 5:2 method.

- While intermittent fasting may lead to weight loss and improved metabolic health, it may not be suitable for everyone and consulting a healthcare professional is advised before adopting this eating pattern.

It's essential to consult with a healthcare provider or registered dietitian before starting any new diet plan to ensure that it aligns with your individual health needs and goals. Additionally, focusing on sustainable lifestyle changes, a balanced diet and regular physical activity is key to achieving long-term weight management and overall well-being.

a. Overview of Popular Diet Plans (e.g., Mediterranean, Ketogenic, Paleo)

Certainly, here is an overview of some popular diet plans, including the Mediterranean, Ketogenic and Paleo diets:

1. Mediterranean Diet:

- Based on the traditional eating patterns of people in countries bordering the Mediterranean Sea.

- Emphasizes the consumption of fruits, vegetables, whole grains, legumes, nuts and olive oil, with moderate consumption of fish and poultry and limited intake of red meat and sweets.

- Known for its emphasis on heart-healthy fats and high intake of plant-based foods, which may contribute to improved cardiovascular health and overall well-being.

2. Ketogenic Diet:

- A high-fat, low-carbohydrate diet designed to induce a metabolic state known as ketosis, in which the body burns fat for energy.

- Promotes the consumption of foods rich in healthy fats, moderate amounts of protein and minimal carbohydrates.

- While the ketogenic diet may lead to rapid weight loss and improved blood sugar control, it may not be suitable for everyone and potential side effects, such as the "keto flu," may occur during the initial adaptation phase.

3. Paleo Diet:

- Based on the presumed dietary patterns of Paleolithic humans, focusing on whole, unprocessed foods similar to what early humans would have eaten, such as lean meats, fish, fruits, vegetables, nuts and seeds.

- Excludes foods that became more prevalent with the advent of agriculture, including grains, legumes, dairy products and processed foods.

- While the Paleo diet may promote weight loss and provide a high intake of nutrient-dense foods, critics highlight potential nutritional deficiencies and the restrictive nature of the diet.

Each of these diet plans has its own set of principles and guidelines and their suitability may vary depending on individual health goals, preferences and lifestyle factors. It's important to consult with a healthcare provider or a registered dietitian before starting any new diet plan to ensure that it aligns with your specific health needs and objectives. Additionally, focusing on a balanced and sustainable approach to eating that emphasizes whole, unprocessed foods and meets individual nutritional requirements is crucial for long-term health and well-being.

b. Analyzing Pros and Cons of Different Dieting Approaches

Analyzing the pros and cons of different dieting approaches can help you make informed decisions about which method may be the most suitable for your individual health and lifestyle needs. Here's a general overview of the pros and cons of several common dieting approaches:

1. Mediterranean Diet:

- Pros: Emphasizes whole, nutrient-dense foods, promotes heart health and is generally sustainable and flexible.

- Cons: May require significant changes in dietary habits and some individuals may find it challenging to limit red meat and processed foods.

2. Ketogenic Diet:

- Pros: Can lead to rapid weight loss, helps control blood sugar levels and may have potential benefits for individuals with certain medical conditions, such as epilepsy.

- Cons: Initial side effects during adaptation (keto flu), restrictive nature may be challenging to maintain long-term and potential risks for individuals with certain health conditions or those on certain medications.

3. Paleo Diet:

- Pros: Focuses on whole, unprocessed foods, encourages high intake of fruits and vegetables and can lead to weight loss and improved overall health in some individuals.

- Cons: Restrictive in terms of certain food groups, potential for nutritional deficiencies and lack of long-term research on its effectiveness and safety.

4. Vegetarian and Vegan Diets:

- Pros: High intake of plant-based foods, potential for improved heart health and reduced risk of chronic diseases and focus on ethical and environmental considerations.

- Cons: Potential for nutrient deficiencies if not properly planned, especially for nutrients like vitamin B12, iron and omega-3 fatty acids and may require careful meal planning to ensure adequate protein intake.

5. DASH Diet:

- Pros: Promotes heart health, emphasizes a balanced diet rich in fruits, vegetables and whole grains and is considered a flexible and sustainable approach to healthy eating.

- Cons: May require adjustments in dietary habits and some individuals may find it challenging to limit sodium intake.

6. Intermittent Fasting:

- Pros: Can simplify meal planning, may lead to weight loss and improved metabolic health and can be flexible and adaptable to various lifestyles.

- Cons: May lead to feelings of hunger and irritability during fasting periods, may not be suitable for everyone and requires careful monitoring to ensure adequate nutrient intake during eating windows.

When considering a specific dieting approach, it's essential to assess its potential benefits and drawbacks in relation to your personal health goals, preferences and any existing health conditions. Consulting with a healthcare provider or a registered dietitian can provide personalized guidance and ensure that you select a dieting approach that aligns with your individual needs and promotes long-term health and well-being.

c. Customizing a Diet Plan Based on Personal Preferences and Lifestyle

Customizing a diet plan based on your personal preferences and lifestyle is key to creating a sustainable and enjoyable eating pattern that supports your health and well-being. Here are some steps to help you tailor a diet plan that aligns with your individual needs and goals:

1. Assess Your Dietary Preferences: Consider the types of foods you enjoy and those you prefer to avoid. Identify your favorite fruits, vegetables, whole grains, lean proteins and healthy fats to incorporate into your meal plan.

2. Set Realistic Goals: Define your health objectives, whether they involve weight management, improved energy levels, or overall well-being. Establish specific, measurable, achievable, relevant and time-bound (SMART) goals to guide your dietary choices.

3. Plan Balanced Meals: Design a meal plan that includes a balance of macronutrients, such as carbohydrates, proteins and fats, to meet your nutritional needs. Incorporate a variety of colorful fruits and vegetables, whole grains and lean sources of protein into your meals.

4. Consider Meal Timing: Determine the meal frequency and timing that best suits your schedule and preferences.

Plan regular meals and snacks throughout the day to maintain energy levels and prevent excessive hunger that can lead to unhealthy food choices.

5. Choose Healthy Cooking Methods: Opt for cooking techniques that preserve the nutritional quality of your foods, such as steaming, grilling, baking, or sautéing with minimal added fats. Experiment with herbs, spices and healthy marinades to enhance the flavors of your meals.

6. Include Snacks and Treats: Integrate nutritious snacks and occasional treats into your diet plan to satisfy cravings and prevent feelings of deprivation. Choose wholesome snack options, such as yogurt with fruits, raw nuts, or vegetable sticks with hummus, to support your overall dietary goals.

7. Stay Hydrated: Ensure adequate hydration by drinking water throughout the day and incorporating hydrating foods like fruits and vegetables into your meals and snacks.

8. Practice Mindful Eating: Focus on mindful eating by paying attention to your hunger and fullness cues, savoring each bite and avoiding distractions during meals. Eat slowly and appreciate the flavors and textures of your food.

9. Adapt to Your Lifestyle: Tailor your diet plan to accommodate your daily routine, work schedule and any dietary restrictions or food allergies you may have. Make adjustments as needed to ensure that your diet plan is manageable and sustainable in the long term.

By customizing your diet plan to reflect your personal preferences and lifestyle, you can create a nourishing and enjoyable eating pattern that supports your overall health and well-being. Consult with a registered dietitian or nutritionist to receive personalized guidance and recommendations that cater to your specific dietary needs, preferences and health objectives.

8. HEALTHY EATING HABITS FOR LONG-TERM MAINTENANCE

Developing healthy eating habits is essential for long-term weight management and overall well-being. Adopting sustainable dietary practices can help you maintain a balanced and nutritious diet while promoting a healthy lifestyle. Here are some key healthy eating habits to incorporate for long-term maintenance:

1. Eat a Variety of Nutrient-Dense Foods: Include a diverse range of fruits, vegetables, whole grains, lean proteins and healthy fats in your diet to ensure you receive a wide spectrum of essential vitamins, minerals and antioxidants.

2. Practice Portion Control: Be mindful of portion sizes to avoid overeating and unnecessary calorie consumption. Use smaller plates and bowls to help manage portion sizes and prevent overindulgence.

3. Emphasize Whole Foods: Choose whole, unprocessed foods over refined and processed options. Whole foods contain higher amounts of nutrients, fiber and beneficial compounds that support overall health and satiety.

4. Stay Hydrated: Drink an adequate amount of water throughout the day to stay hydrated and support overall

bodily functions. Adequate hydration is crucial for maintaining energy levels and promoting optimal physical and cognitive performance.

5. Limit Added Sugars and Processed Foods: Reduce your intake of added sugars, sugary beverages and processed snacks, as they can contribute to weight gain and various health issues. Instead, opt for whole fruits and healthier snack alternatives.

6. Cook at Home: Prepare meals at home as much as possible to have better control over the ingredients and cooking methods. Home-cooked meals are generally healthier than restaurant or takeout options.

7. Read Food Labels: Pay attention to food labels and ingredient lists to make informed choices about the products you consume. Choose foods with minimal added sugars, unhealthy fats and artificial ingredients.

8. Plan and Prep Meals: Plan your meals in advance and consider meal prepping to ensure that you have healthy options readily available. This can help you avoid the temptation of unhealthy convenience foods and make it easier to stick to your healthy eating plan.

9. Moderation is Key: Practice moderation in your eating habits, including portion sizes, indulgences and treats. Avoid restrictive diets that may lead to feelings of deprivation and instead focus on creating a balanced and sustainable approach to eating.

10. Enjoy Meals Mindfully: Practice mindful eating by savoring each bite, chewing slowly and paying attention to hunger and fullness cues. Eating mindfully can help you appreciate food more and prevent overeating.

Incorporating these healthy eating habits into your daily routine can support your long-term maintenance of a healthy weight and overall well-being. Remember that small, consistent changes can lead to significant improvements over time. If you need further guidance or personalized advice, consult with a registered dietitian or nutritionist to develop a customized eating plan that aligns with your specific dietary preferences, lifestyle and health goals.

a. Importance of Building Sustainable Habits

Building sustainable habits is crucial for long-term success in maintaining a healthy lifestyle, achieving personal goals and promoting overall well-being. Sustainable habits are those that can be maintained consistently over time, leading to lasting positive changes in various aspects of life. Here's why building sustainable habits is important:

1. Long-Term Health and Well-Being: Sustainable habits contribute to improved physical and mental health, promoting overall well-being and reducing the risk of chronic diseases associated with poor lifestyle choices.

2. Consistent Progress and Results: By integrating sustainable habits into your daily routine, you can make steady progress toward your goals, whether they relate to weight management, fitness, or overall personal development.

3. Stress Reduction and Improved Mental Health: Establishing sustainable habits can help reduce stress, increase resilience and improve mental health. Consistent healthy behaviors can positively impact mood, cognition and emotional well-being.

4. Increased Energy and Vitality: Sustainable habits, such as regular exercise, balanced nutrition and adequate sleep, can

boost energy levels and enhance overall vitality, leading to improved productivity and a better quality of life.

5. Enhanced Self-Discipline and Self-Efficacy: Practicing sustainable habits fosters self-discipline and self-efficacy, helping you develop a sense of control over your actions and outcomes. This can lead to increased confidence and motivation to pursue further personal growth and development.

6. Prevention of Yo-Yo Dieting and Unhealthy Behaviors: Sustainable habits promote a balanced and consistent approach to health and wellness, reducing the likelihood of yo-yo dieting, extreme exercise regimens and other unhealthy behaviors that can have negative consequences on physical and emotional well-being.

7. Improved Resilience to Setbacks: Sustainable habits cultivate resilience, enabling you to bounce back from setbacks and challenges more effectively. This resilience allows you to maintain a positive mindset and continue working toward your goals despite obstacles or temporary lapses.

8. Positive Impact on Relationships: Sustainable habits can positively impact your relationships with others, as they

may inspire and motivate those around you to adopt healthier and more sustainable lifestyle choices.

By focusing on building sustainable habits, you can create a solid foundation for lasting personal growth and development. Start with small, manageable changes and gradually incorporate new habits into your daily routine to promote a healthier and more fulfilling lifestyle. Remember that consistency and persistence are key to achieving long-term success and maintaining a positive and balanced approach to overall well-being.

b. Mindful Eating for Weight Maintenance

Mindful eating is a powerful practice that can support weight maintenance by promoting a healthy relationship with food, preventing overeating and enhancing overall well-being. By incorporating mindful eating principles into your daily routine, you can develop a greater awareness of your body's hunger and fullness cues, leading to more balanced and sustainable eating habits. Here are some mindful eating strategies specifically beneficial for weight maintenance:

1. Eat Slowly and Mindfully: Take your time to savor each bite and chew your food thoroughly. Pay attention to the flavors, textures and aromas of your meals, allowing yourself to fully enjoy the eating experience.

2. Listen to Your Body: Tune into your body's hunger and fullness signals to identify when you're truly hungry and when you've had enough to eat. Stop eating before you feel overly full and avoid mindless snacking or emotional eating.

3. Eliminate Distractions: Minimize distractions, such as television, electronic devices, or work-related activities, during meal times. Create a calm and peaceful eating environment that allows you to focus solely on the act of eating and enjoying your food.

4. Engage Your Senses: Engage all your senses while eating, paying attention to the colors, smells, textures and sounds of your food. This can help you feel more connected to your meals and appreciate the sensory experience of eating.

5. Practice Portion Control: Be mindful of portion sizes and serve yourself appropriate amounts of food. Use smaller plates and bowls to help control portion sizes and prevent overeating.

6. Distinguish Physical Hunger from Emotional Hunger: Learn to differentiate between physical hunger and emotional triggers that may lead to overeating. Find alternative ways to manage stress and emotions, such as engaging in physical activity, practicing relaxation techniques, or seeking social support.

7. Savor Balanced and Nutrient-Dense Meals: Focus on consuming balanced meals that include a variety of nutrient-dense foods, such as fruits, vegetables, whole grains, lean proteins and healthy fats. Prioritize the nutritional quality of your meals to support your overall health and well-being.

By cultivating mindful eating habits, you can develop a more conscious and balanced approach to food, leading to improved satisfaction with meals, better digestion and enhanced self-awareness around your dietary choices. Mindful eating can be a valuable tool for weight maintenance, helping you establish a healthier relationship with food and achieve a more sustainable and balanced lifestyle.

c. Avoiding Weight Regain and Plateaus

Avoiding weight regain and plateaus is crucial for maintaining long-term weight loss success. Here are some effective strategies to help prevent weight regain and overcome plateaus:

1. Sustainable Lifestyle Changes: Focus on adopting sustainable lifestyle changes rather than temporary dieting. Implement long-term habits that promote balanced nutrition, regular physical activity and healthy coping mechanisms for managing stress and emotions.

2. Regular Physical Activity: Incorporate a combination of cardiovascular exercises, strength training and flexibility exercises into your routine. Vary your workouts to prevent boredom and continuously challenge your body.

3. Monitor Your Progress: Keep track of your food intake, exercise routine and weight fluctuations to identify any patterns or potential challenges. Regular monitoring can help you stay accountable and make necessary adjustments to your lifestyle.

4. Set Realistic Goals: Establish achievable and realistic weight loss and maintenance goals. Avoid setting overly ambitious targets that may lead to frustration and an increased likelihood of abandoning your efforts.

5. Diversify Your Diet: Incorporate a variety of nutrient-dense foods into your meals to ensure you're receiving a wide spectrum of essential vitamins and minerals. Experiment with new recipes and ingredients to keep your meals interesting and satisfying.

6. Practice Mindful Eating: Develop mindful eating habits to help you become more aware of your hunger and fullness cues. Pay attention to your body's signals to prevent overeating and emotional eating.

7. Adjust Your Caloric Intake: Reassess your caloric needs periodically and adjust your intake based on changes in your weight and activity levels. Consult with a registered dietitian to determine an appropriate calorie range for weight maintenance.

8. Manage Stress and Emotional Eating: Find healthy and effective strategies to manage stress and emotions, such as practicing mindfulness, engaging in physical activities you enjoy, or seeking support from friends and family.

9. Regularly Reassess Your Plan: Regularly review and reassess your weight loss and maintenance plan to ensure it continues to align with your current goals and lifestyle.

Make necessary modifications to your diet and exercise regimen as needed.

10. Seek Professional Support: Consult with a healthcare provider, registered dietitian, or certified fitness professional for personalized guidance and support. They can provide expert advice tailored to your specific needs and help you navigate any challenges you may encounter.

By implementing these strategies, you can maintain your weight loss achievements, overcome plateaus and establish a healthy and balanced lifestyle that supports long-term weight management and overall well-being.

9. SPECIAL CONSIDERATIONS FOR WEIGHT LOSS

When embarking on a weight loss journey, it's essential to consider various factors that can influence your approach and success. Here are some special considerations to keep in mind:

1. Underlying Health Conditions: If you have any underlying health conditions, such as diabetes, hypertension, or hormonal imbalances, consult a healthcare professional before starting any weight loss program. They can provide guidance on the most appropriate approach for your specific health needs.

2. Medication and Supplements: Certain medications or supplements may affect your weight or interact with specific dietary interventions. Discuss any medications or supplements you're taking with your healthcare provider to ensure they align with your weight loss goals.

3. Metabolic Rate and Hormonal Changes: Individual variations in metabolic rate and hormonal changes can influence weight loss. Factors such as age, gender and medical history can impact how your body responds to different diet and exercise regimens.

4. Emotional and Psychological Factors: Emotional and psychological factors, including stress, anxiety and depression, can significantly impact eating behaviors and weight management. Addressing these factors through counseling, therapy, or stress-reduction techniques can support a more holistic approach to weight loss.

5. Dietary Preferences and Cultural Considerations: Personal dietary preferences and cultural considerations can play a significant role in adherence to a weight loss plan. Consider incorporating traditional foods and dishes that align with your cultural background while focusing on balanced nutrition and portion control.

6. Body Image and Self-Esteem: Developing a positive body image and nurturing self-esteem are essential for a healthy relationship with food and sustainable weight management. Focus on overall well-being and self-acceptance rather than pursuing an unrealistic or unhealthy body ideal.

7. Physical Activity Limitations: If you have physical limitations or chronic pain, consult with a healthcare provider or a certified fitness professional to identify suitable exercise options that accommodate your abilities and promote physical well-being.

8. Sleep and Stress Management: Prioritize adequate sleep and effective stress management strategies to support healthy weight loss. Lack of sleep and chronic stress can negatively impact hormonal balance, appetite regulation and overall well-being, hindering your weight loss efforts.

9. Support System and Accountability: Establish a support system with friends, family, or a support group to provide encouragement and accountability throughout your weight loss journey. Share your goals with others who can offer motivation, guidance and positive reinforcement.

By considering these factors and addressing any specific considerations related to your health and well-being, you can develop a comprehensive approach to weight loss that is tailored to your individual needs and promotes a sustainable and holistic path to achieving your goals.

a. Weight Loss and Age-Related Considerations

Weight loss can present unique considerations based on age-related factors. As individuals age, physiological changes, lifestyle adjustments and health considerations can influence the approach to weight loss. Here are some age-related considerations to keep in mind:

1. Metabolic Rate Changes: Metabolism tends to naturally slow down with age, making weight loss more challenging. To counteract this, focus on incorporating regular physical activity and strength training exercises to help maintain muscle mass and support a healthy metabolic rate.

2. Nutritional Needs: Nutritional requirements may shift with age, requiring adjustments in dietary intake to accommodate changes in metabolism and energy expenditure. Ensure your diet includes nutrient-dense foods that provide essential vitamins, minerals and adequate protein for maintaining muscle mass and bone health.

3. Hormonal Changes: Hormonal fluctuations, particularly in menopause for women, can influence weight distribution and metabolism. Consult with a healthcare provider to address any specific concerns related to hormonal changes and to explore appropriate strategies for managing weight during this stage of life.

4. Bone Health and Muscle Mass: Focus on activities that support bone health, such as weight-bearing exercises and resistance training, to help prevent age-related muscle loss and osteoporosis. Adequate protein intake is also important for preserving muscle mass and supporting overall physical function.

5. Joint Health and Mobility: Aging can bring about joint stiffness and reduced mobility, impacting the ability to engage in certain forms of physical activity. Choose low-impact exercises, such as swimming, yoga, or walking, to minimize stress on the joints while maintaining an active lifestyle.

6. Chronic Health Conditions: The presence of chronic health conditions, such as cardiovascular disease, diabetes, or arthritis, may require specific dietary and exercise modifications. Work with a healthcare provider to develop a comprehensive weight loss plan that considers any preexisting health conditions and promotes overall well-being.

7. Cognitive Health and Emotional Well-Being: Pay attention to cognitive health and emotional well-being, as these aspects can significantly impact eating behaviors and adherence to a weight loss program. Incorporate activities

that support mental agility and stress management, such as mindfulness practices and social engagement.

By acknowledging these age-related considerations and tailoring your weight loss approach accordingly, you can develop a comprehensive and sustainable plan that supports overall health and well-being throughout the aging process. Consult with a healthcare provider or a registered dietitian to receive personalized guidance and recommendations that address your specific age-related needs and goals.

b. Managing Weight Loss with Medical Conditions

Managing weight loss with certain medical conditions requires careful consideration and often involves a personalized approach that accounts for the specific health concerns and needs of the individual. Here are some general guidelines for managing weight loss with certain medical conditions:

1. Diabetes: For individuals with diabetes, it is essential to monitor blood sugar levels and choose foods that have a minimal impact on blood glucose. Focus on consuming a balanced diet that includes complex carbohydrates, lean proteins and healthy fats. Coordinate with a healthcare provider or a registered dietitian to develop a meal plan that supports blood sugar control and weight management.

2. Cardiovascular Disease: Individuals with cardiovascular disease should prioritize a heart-healthy diet that includes plenty of fruits, vegetables, whole grains and lean proteins while limiting saturated and trans fats, sodium and added sugars. Incorporate regular physical activity, as approved by a healthcare provider, to support heart health and overall well-being.

3. Hypertension: To manage weight loss with hypertension, emphasize a diet rich in fruits, vegetables, whole grains and low-fat dairy products while minimizing sodium intake. Engage in regular aerobic exercise and incorporate stress-

reduction techniques to help lower blood pressure and support overall cardiovascular health.

4. Thyroid Disorders: Individuals with thyroid disorders may experience fluctuations in metabolism and weight. Work closely with a healthcare provider to adjust medication as needed and to develop a comprehensive weight management plan that supports thyroid function. Focus on consuming a balanced diet that includes foods rich in iodine, selenium and other essential nutrients for thyroid health.

5. Gastrointestinal Disorders: Gastrointestinal disorders, such as irritable bowel syndrome (IBS) or inflammatory bowel disease (IBD), may require dietary modifications to manage symptoms and support healthy digestion. Work with a healthcare provider or a registered dietitian to identify trigger foods and develop a meal plan that minimizes gastrointestinal distress while promoting weight loss and overall well-being.

6. Chronic Pain or Mobility Issues: Individuals with chronic pain or mobility issues should focus on low-impact physical activities and exercises that are gentle on the joints. Consult with a healthcare provider or a physical therapist to identify suitable exercises that support weight loss without exacerbating pain or discomfort.

Always consult with a healthcare provider before implementing any weight loss plan, especially if you have a preexisting medical condition. A healthcare provider or a registered dietitian can provide personalized guidance and recommendations tailored to your specific health needs and goals, ensuring a safe and effective approach to managing weight loss while addressing any underlying medical concerns.

c. Tips for Overcoming Weight Loss Plateaus

Overcoming weight loss plateaus can be challenging, but with the right strategies and adjustments, you can jumpstart your progress and continue working toward your goals. Here are some effective tips for overcoming weight loss plateaus:

1. Review Your Eating Habits: Assess your current dietary intake and ensure that you're maintaining a calorie deficit by consuming nutrient-dense, whole foods. Avoid mindless snacking and monitor portion sizes to prevent overeating.

2. Adjust Your Exercise Routine: Vary your workout intensity, duration and type of exercises to challenge your body and prevent adaptation. Incorporate strength training to build lean muscle mass, which can help boost metabolism and support continued weight loss.

3. Increase Physical Activity: Increase your overall physical activity throughout the day by incorporating more movement, such as taking short walks, using the stairs, or participating in active hobbies. Aim for at least 150 minutes of moderate-intensity aerobic activity per week.

4. Modify Your Caloric Intake: Adjust your calorie intake by reducing portion sizes slightly or incorporating more low-calorie, nutrient-dense foods into your meals. Be

cautious not to lower your calorie intake too drastically, as this can slow down your metabolism and hinder weight loss progress.

5. Stay Hydrated: Drink an adequate amount of water throughout the day to stay hydrated and support your body's metabolic processes. Sometimes, thirst can be mistaken for hunger, leading to unnecessary calorie consumption.

6. Manage Stress Levels: Practice stress-reduction techniques, such as meditation, yoga, or deep breathing exercises, to manage cortisol levels and prevent stress-related weight gain. Chronic stress can contribute to weight loss plateaus, so prioritizing stress management is essential.

7. Get Sufficient Sleep: Aim for at least 7-9 hours of quality sleep each night to support overall health and well-being. Inadequate sleep can disrupt hormonal balance, leading to increased appetite and decreased energy levels, which may hinder weight loss efforts.

8. Reassess Your Goals: Reevaluate your weight loss goals to ensure they are realistic and attainable. Set new short-term and long-term goals to maintain motivation and focus on the progress you've made rather than fixating on the scale.

9. Monitor Non-Scale Victories: Focus on non-scale victories, such as improvements in energy levels, increased strength, or better-fitting clothes. Acknowledging these achievements can help boost motivation and reinforce positive lifestyle changes.

10. Seek Support and Accountability: Enlist the support of friends, family, or a support group to provide encouragement and accountability. Share your challenges and successes with others who can offer motivation and guidance throughout your weight loss journey.

By implementing these strategies, you can overcome weight loss plateaus and continue making progress toward your goals. Remember that consistency, patience and a holistic approach to health and well-being are key to achieving sustainable weight loss and overall wellness.

10. FREQUENTLY ASKED QUESTIONS ABOUT WEIGHT LOSS AND NUTRITION

1. What is the best diet for weight loss?

- There is no one-size-fits-all answer, as the best diet for weight loss varies depending on individual preferences, lifestyle and health considerations. It's essential to focus on a balanced and sustainable eating plan that includes a variety of nutrient-dense foods and suits your specific dietary needs and goals.

2. How many calories should I consume to lose weight?

- The number of calories needed for weight loss varies from person to person and depends on factors such as age, gender, weight, height and activity level. Consult with a healthcare provider or a registered dietitian to determine an appropriate calorie range that supports healthy and sustainable weight loss.

3. Is exercise necessary for weight loss?

- While diet plays a significant role in weight loss, regular physical activity is essential for overall health and can complement your weight loss efforts. Exercise helps increase calorie expenditure, build muscle mass and improve overall fitness, contributing to sustainable weight management.

4. What are some healthy snacks for weight loss?

- Healthy snack options for weight loss include fruits, vegetables with hummus or Greek yogurt dip, nuts, seeds, whole-grain crackers and low-fat cheese. Choosing nutrient-dense snacks that provide a balance of carbohydrates, protein and healthy fats can help keep you satisfied and prevent overeating.

5. Can I lose weight without feeling hungry all the time?

- Yes, you can lose weight without feeling hungry by choosing nutrient-dense foods that are high in fiber and protein, which can help promote satiety. Incorporating healthy fats and staying hydrated can also help you feel more satisfied and prevent excessive hunger.

6. Are there any supplements that can aid in weight loss?

- While certain supplements may claim to aid in weight loss, it's essential to approach them with caution and consult with a healthcare provider before incorporating them into your regimen. Focus on obtaining essential nutrients from whole foods and consider discussing potential supplementation with a healthcare professional if necessary.

7. How can I maintain my weight loss after reaching my goal?

- Maintaining weight loss involves practicing sustainable lifestyle habits, including regular physical activity, mindful eating and a balanced diet. Focus on long-term behavior changes, monitor your progress and continue to prioritize your overall health and well-being.

These answers provide general guidance, but it's essential to consult with a healthcare provider or a registered dietitian for personalized advice tailored to your specific health needs and goals.

a. Addressing Common Myths and Misconceptions

Certainly, here are some common myths and misconceptions related to weight loss and nutrition, along with the facts that can help dispel these misconceptions:

1. Myth: Skipping meals can help with weight loss.

- Fact: Skipping meals can lead to overeating later in the day and can disrupt your metabolism. It's important to eat regular, balanced meals to support healthy weight management.

2. Myth: All fats are unhealthy and should be avoided.

- Fact: Healthy fats, such as those found in avocados, nuts, seeds and fatty fish, are essential for overall health and can even support weight loss when consumed in moderation. They provide important nutrients and can help you feel full and satisfied.

3. Myth: Carbohydrates should be completely eliminated for effective weight loss.

- Fact: Carbohydrates are an important energy source for the body. Choosing complex carbohydrates, such as whole grains, fruits and vegetables, can provide essential nutrients and fiber while supporting sustainable weight loss.

4. Myth: All calories are equal, regardless of the source.

- Fact: The source of calories matters, as different foods can have varying effects on hunger, metabolism and overall health. Nutrient-dense foods that are high in fiber and protein can help keep you full and satisfied, supporting your weight loss efforts.

5. Myth: Weight loss supplements can provide a quick fix for shedding pounds.

- Fact: Many weight loss supplements are not regulated and may have limited scientific evidence supporting their effectiveness. Sustainable weight loss is best achieved through a balanced diet, regular physical activity and healthy lifestyle habits.

6. Myth: Eating after 8 p.m. will lead to weight gain.

- Fact: The timing of meals does not directly impact weight gain. What matters more is the overall calorie intake and the quality of the foods you consume throughout the day. Focus on balanced meals and snacks, regardless of the time of day.

7. Myth: Exercise alone is enough to lose weight.

- Fact: While exercise is crucial for overall health, sustainable weight loss is best achieved through a combination of regular physical activity and a balanced diet. Creating a calorie deficit through a combination of exercise and dietary changes is key to effective weight loss.

It's important to consult with a healthcare provider or a registered dietitian to receive accurate and personalized information that aligns with your specific health needs and goals. By understanding these common myths and misconceptions, you can make informed decisions about your diet and lifestyle to support long-term health and well-being.

b. Tips for Sustaining Motivation and Consistency

Maintaining motivation and consistency is key to achieving long-term success in any endeavor, including weight loss and nutrition. Here are some effective tips to help you sustain motivation and consistency:

1. Set Realistic Goals: Establish achievable and realistic goals that are specific, measurable and time-bound. Break down larger goals into smaller milestones to track your progress and stay motivated.

2. Find Intrinsic Motivation: Identify your personal reasons for wanting to achieve your goals. Connect with the deeper meaning behind your aspirations to help fuel your motivation from within.

3. Celebrate Small Wins: Acknowledge and celebrate your achievements, no matter how small. Recognizing your progress can boost your confidence and provide the momentum you need to keep moving forward.

4. Create a Supportive Environment: Surround yourself with individuals who support your goals and encourage your progress. Engage with like-minded individuals, join support groups, or enlist the help of a fitness buddy to stay motivated and accountable.

5. Develop Consistent Habits: Establish consistent daily habits that align with your goals. Whether it's meal prepping, scheduling regular workouts, or practicing mindfulness, integrating these habits into your routine can foster a sense of structure and commitment.

6. Practice Self-Compassion: Be kind to yourself and recognize that setbacks are a natural part of any journey. Approach challenges with self-compassion, learn from any obstacles and use them as opportunities for growth and improvement.

7. Stay Educated and Informed: Continuously educate yourself about nutrition, exercise and overall well-being. Stay informed about the latest research and evidence-based practices to make informed decisions that support your health and fitness goals.

8. Visualize Success: Create a clear mental image of what success looks like for you. Visualize yourself achieving your goals and experiencing the positive outcomes that come with your hard work and dedication.

9. Practice Mindfulness and Stress Reduction: Engage in activities that promote mindfulness and reduce stress, such as meditation, yoga, or deep breathing exercises. Managing

stress can help you stay focused, positive and motivated throughout your journey.

10. Reassess and Adjust: Regularly reassess your goals and strategies to ensure they continue to align with your evolving needs and priorities. Make necessary adjustments to your approach to keep your motivation high and maintain consistency in your efforts.

By incorporating these tips into your daily routine, you can foster sustainable motivation and consistency, helping you stay on track toward achieving your weight loss and nutrition goals.

11. CONCLUSION: EMBRACING A HEALTHY LIFESTYLE FOR LASTING RESULTS

In conclusion, embracing a healthy lifestyle is essential for achieving lasting results in weight management and overall well-being. By prioritizing balanced nutrition, regular physical activity and mindful living, you can establish sustainable habits that promote long-term health and vitality. Remember that small, consistent changes can lead to significant improvements over time and that adopting a holistic approach to wellness can contribute to a more fulfilling and enriching life.

Continue to prioritize your physical and mental health and approach your journey with patience, self-compassion and a growth-oriented mindset. Seek support from healthcare professionals, nutrition experts and a strong support network to guide you along the way. Embrace the journey as an opportunity for self-discovery, personal growth and the cultivation of a positive relationship with your body and food.

By making informed choices, practicing self-care and maintaining a positive outlook, you can create a foundation for a healthy lifestyle that extends far beyond weight management. Stay committed to your goals, stay curious and remain open to new possibilities for enhancing your well-being. Here's to your continued success and a life of vibrant health and happiness.

a. Celebrating Non-Scale Victories and Progress

Celebrating non-scale victories and progress is a wonderful way to acknowledge your achievements beyond just the number on the scale. Non-scale victories encompass various positive changes that contribute to your overall well-being and quality of life. Here are some non-scale victories worth celebrating:

1. Improved Energy Levels: Recognize and celebrate any increase in your energy levels and overall vitality, which may result from your healthier lifestyle choices and improved nutrition.

2. Enhanced Mood and Mental Well-Being: Acknowledge any improvements in your mood, reduced stress levels and enhanced mental clarity that may have resulted from regular physical activity and a balanced diet.

3. Better Sleep Quality: Celebrate any positive changes in your sleep patterns, such as improved sleep quality, better sleep duration and a more consistent sleep schedule, which can positively impact your overall health and well-being.

4. Increased Strength and Endurance: Take pride in any advancements in your physical strength, endurance and stamina, whether it's lifting heavier weights, completing more repetitions, or achieving new fitness milestones.

5. Clothing Fit and Comfort: Celebrate any noticeable changes in the way your clothes fit and feel, as this can be a clear indication of positive changes in your body composition and overall fitness level.

6. Healthy Habits Formation: Recognize the establishment of healthier habits, such as meal planning, regular exercise routines, mindful eating practices and stress management techniques, which contribute to a sustainable and balanced lifestyle.

7. Body Confidence and Self-Esteem: Embrace any improvements in your body confidence and self-esteem, acknowledging your progress in cultivating a positive body image and fostering a healthy relationship with your body.

8. Positive Feedback from Others: Acknowledge any positive feedback or encouragement you receive from friends, family, or healthcare professionals who recognize and appreciate your commitment to improving your health and well-being.

By celebrating these non-scale victories, you can reinforce your progress, boost your motivation and cultivate a sense of accomplishment that extends beyond numerical measurements. Embrace the journey and continue to prioritize your overall health and happiness.

b. Committing to Long-Term Health and Wellness

Committing to long-term health and wellness is a significant investment in your overall well-being and quality of life. By prioritizing sustainable lifestyle practices and fostering a holistic approach to health, you can establish a solid foundation for lasting vitality and fulfillment. Here are some essential principles to consider when committing to long-term health and wellness:

1. Consistent Self-Care: Make self-care a priority by engaging in activities that nurture your physical, mental and emotional well-being. Set aside time for relaxation, stress management and activities that bring you joy and fulfillment.

2. Balanced Nutrition: Emphasize a balanced and varied diet that includes a diverse range of nutrient-dense foods, such as fruits, vegetables, whole grains, lean proteins and healthy fats. Prioritize portion control and mindful eating to support your overall health and weight management goals.

3. Regular Physical Activity: Incorporate regular physical activity into your routine, including a combination of cardiovascular exercises, strength training and flexibility exercises. Find activities you enjoy to help promote consistency and long-term adherence.

4. Quality Sleep: Prioritize quality sleep by establishing a consistent sleep schedule and creating a relaxing sleep environment. Aim for 7-9 hours of restful sleep each night to support overall health, cognitive function and emotional well-being.

5. Stress Management: Implement effective stress management techniques, such as meditation, deep breathing exercises, or engaging in hobbies and activities that bring you a sense of calm and relaxation. Managing stress is crucial for maintaining overall health and preventing the onset of stress-related health issues.

6. Regular Health Screenings: Schedule regular health check-ups and screenings to monitor your overall health and detect any potential health concerns at an early stage. Stay proactive in managing your health by following the recommendations of healthcare professionals.

7. Social Connections: Cultivate and maintain meaningful social connections with friends, family and community members. Engage in social activities that promote a sense of belonging, support and companionship, as strong social connections can positively impact your overall well-being.

8. Lifelong Learning: Foster a mindset of continuous learning and personal growth by seeking new knowledge, exploring new interests and challenging yourself intellectually. Embrace opportunities for personal development and self-improvement to enhance your overall quality of life.

By embracing these principles and incorporating them into your daily life, you can establish a sustainable and comprehensive approach to long-term health and wellness. Remember that small, consistent steps can lead to significant improvements over time, contributing to a fulfilling and vibrant life.

c. Resources for Ongoing Support and Guidance

To continue your journey toward improved health and wellness, consider exploring the following resources for ongoing support and guidance:

1. Healthcare Professionals: Consult with your primary care physician, registered dietitian, or certified fitness trainer for personalized guidance and support tailored to your specific health needs and goals.

2. Nutrition and Wellness Apps: Explore reputable nutrition and wellness apps that can help you track your food intake, monitor your physical activity and provide valuable insights into your progress and habits.

3. Online Communities and Support Groups: Join online communities and support groups focused on health, fitness and nutrition. Engage with like-minded individuals, share experiences and receive encouragement and advice from a supportive network.

4. Health and Wellness Websites: Visit reputable health and wellness websites that provide evidence-based information on nutrition, fitness and overall well-being. Look for resources backed by credible sources and medical professionals.

5. Books and Publications: Explore a variety of books, journals and publications written by experts in the fields of nutrition, health and fitness. Look for reputable authors and publications that offer practical advice and strategies for maintaining a healthy lifestyle.

6. Fitness Classes and Workshops: Attend local fitness classes, workshops, or seminars that focus on various aspects of health and wellness. Participate in educational sessions, hands-on activities and group exercises to enhance your knowledge and skills.

7. Wellness Coaching Programs: Consider enrolling in wellness coaching programs that provide personalized guidance, accountability and support for achieving your health and wellness goals. Work with experienced coaches who can help you develop sustainable lifestyle habits and overcome any challenges you may encounter.

8. Corporate Wellness Programs: If available, explore corporate wellness programs offered by your employer. Take advantage of wellness initiatives, resources and activities that promote a healthy work-life balance and support your overall well-being.